Essential Oil Recipes For Healthy Living

A Guide For Natural Living Using Essential Oils

Disclaimer and Terms of Use:

Effort has been made to ensure that the information in this book is accurate and complete, however, the author and the publisher do not warrant the accuracy of the information, text and graphics contained within the book due to the rapidly changing nature of science, research, known and unknown facts and internet. The Author and the publisher do not hold any responsibility for errors, omissions or contrary interpretation of the subject matter herein. This book is presented solely for motivational and informational purposes only.

Table of Contents

Chapter 1   Essential Oil Recipes For Health

Essential oils have been used for the relief of various ailments since the time of our ancestors. Below are some essential oil blends for various ailments.

High Blood Pressure Blend

Ingredients:

1 oz. Carrier Oil of your choice

10 drops Ylang Ylang Essential Oil

5 drops Cypress Essential Oil

5 drops Marjoram Essential Oil

Directions:

1. Combine essential oils and transfer in a glass container.

2. Place a few drops on your palms and rub oil mixture on the heart and on your left foot and left hand. These are the reflexology points of the heart. Doing so will help regulate your blood flow.

Scar Vanishing Blend

Ingredients:

6 drops Myrrh

6 drops Helichrysm

4 drops Lavender

2 drops Sandalwood

1 oz. Carrier oil of your choice

Directions:

Combine essential oils and massage on new scar twice daily; once after morning bath and before going to sleep at night.

Headache Reliever

Ingredients:

  5 ml Fractionated Coconut Oil (FCO)

  10 drops Frankincense

  10 drops Birch

  10 drops Wintergreen

  30 drops Peppermint

  30 drops Lavender

Directions:

Rub Essential Oils mixture on your forehead, temples, brain stem and at the back of your neck. Apply as needed.

Colds Reliever For Kids

Ingredients:

 1 drop Thyme combined with Linalol

 3 drops Lavender EO

 5 drops Tea Tree EO

 10 drops Ravensara

 10 drops Eucalyptus EO

Directions:

Dilute the colds reliever mix in vegetable oil before adding it in your child's bath.

For babies (2-18 months) – 1 drop colds reliever mixed in 1 teaspoon vegetable oil.

For toddlers (19 months to 3 years old) – 2 drops colds reliever mixed in 1 teaspoon vegetable oil

For kids (3 to 6 years old) – 3 drops colds reliever mixed in 1 teaspoon vegetable oil

For big kids (7 to 11 years old) – 4 drops colds reliever mixed in 1 teaspoon vegetable oil

For Older kids (12 years old and above) – 5 drops colds reliever mixed in 1 teaspoon vegetable oil.

For kids 3 to 12 years old and older, you may put 2 drops of colds reliever in a cotton or tissue and let the child sniff from it. This will help relieve the symptoms.

*The bath should use warm water but not too warm for babies. At least warm enough that is bearable for the kid.

Labor Aromatherapy Formula for Diffuser

Ingredients:

    20 drops Basil

    42 drops Ylang Ylang

    100 drops Sage

    120 drops Pine

Directions:

Place in diffuser. Enjoy the relaxing scent of this blend. You may use this blend everyday to keep you relaxed.

Regeneration and Pain Relief Blend

Ingredients:

20 drops Marjoram

20 drops Lemongrass

15 drops Deep Blue

10 drops Lavender

10 drops Cypress

10 drops Sandalwood

3 ounces FCO

Directions:

This blend is great for injuries, ligament or tendon damage, cartilage regeneration, and muscle pain. Massage a small amount on the affected area. Use as necessary. Combine the mixture in a roller bottle for easier application.

ADHD/ADD And Anxiety Relief

Ingredients:

  10 drops Marjoram

  15 drops Clary Sage

  20 drops Frankincense

  30 drops Ylang Ylang

  30 drops Lavender

  85 drops Vetiver

  35 drops Coconut oil or

  75 drops Fractionated Coconut Oil (FCO)

Directions:

Apply at the bottom of your feet or your kid's feet before bedtime. At daytime, roll some on your wrists so you can breathe on the scent. You may also put 2 drops of this blend in a tissue so the child can sniff from it. Use as needed.

Jet Lag Relieving Essential Oils

Ingredients:

    5 drops Lavender

    10 drops Black Spruce

    10 drops Orange

    1 oz Jojoba Oil

Directions:

Place a few drops on your palm and rub them together. Breathe on your palm slowly. You will feel relief in a few minutes.

Fertility Blend For Males

Ingredients:

2 drops Lavender

8 drops Whisper EO

10 drops Aromatouch EO

10 drops Basil

10 drops Balance

15 drops Marjoram

15 drops Geranium

25 drops Clary Sage

Directions:

Rub on your palms and breathe in the scent. You may also place a few drops on tissue paper and inhale. Use in the morning and in the evening before going to sleep.

Fertility Blend For Females

Ingredients:

2 drops Lavender

5 drops Eucalyptus

8 drops Elevatation

10 drops Basil

10 drops Aromatouch

15 drops Geranium

15 drops Marjoram

Directions:

Same as the male version: Rub on palms and then breathe in the scent. You may also place a couple of drops on tissue paper and take in the scent. Use in the morning and before going to sleep.

Trauma Relieving Blend

Ingredients:

    5 drops Rose EO

    6 drops Tsuga

    10 drops Spruce

    12 drops Cedarwood

    15 drops Frankincense

    16 drops Lavender

    20 drops Kefir Lime

    20 drops Davana

Directions:

Mix all essential oils in a glass container. Rub a few drops on your palms and inhale on the scent. You may also rub some on your wrist so you can sniff on the scent anytime. Use as needed.

Stress Reducing Essential Oil Blend

Ingredients:

  5 drops Cistus EO

  10 drops Tangerine EO

  20 drops Chamomile EO

  30 drops Lavender EO

Directions:

Mix in carrier oil and rub on your palms and breathe on the sent or place a few drops on a cotton and place under your pillow before sleeping. You may also place a few drops on a tissue or hanky so may sniff on it as needed.

Better Sleep Essential Oil Blends

Ingredients:

5 drops Clary Sage

5 drops Bergamot

10 drops Chamomile

Directions:

Add 2 to 3 drops of the mixture in a tissue and place under your pillow. You may also diffuse by using a drop of Clary Sage, a drop of Bergamot and 2 drops of Chamomile.

OR

Ingredients:

20 drops Lavender

7 drops Vetiver (diluted)

1 oz FCO

Directions:

Place mixture in roller bottle and apply on feet before sleeping at night.

OR

Ingredients:

3 drops Marjoram

1 drop Vetiver

Directions:

Place in diffuser and enjoy a relaxing sleep at night.

OR

Ingredients:

2 drops Nutmeg EO

2 drops Ravensara

2 drops Geranium

Directions:

Diffuse and enjoy its relaxing scent for a good night sleep.

OR

Ingredients:

2 drops Balance

2 drops Serenity

2 drops Frankincense

2 drops Vetiver

1 drop Lavender

Directions:

Diffuse and feel relaxed and energized the next day.

Chapter 2   Essential Oil Recipes For Beauty

Essential oils are also commonly used for beauty products due to their calming and rejuvenating properties. Below are essential oil recipes for beauty you can do at home.

Lavender Honey Lip Balm

Ingredients:

   1 tablespoon Sweet Almond Oil

   1 tablespoon Shea Butter

   2 tablespoons Coconut Oil

   2 tablespoons Beeswax

   ½ teaspoon Raw Honey

   5 drops Frankincense

   15 drops Lavender Essential Oil

Directions:

1. Melt Shea butter, coconut oil and beeswax in a glass bowl placed in a pot of simmering water or use a double broiler of you have one.

2. Remove from heat and stir in sweet almond oil and the essential oils.

3. Place in small containers before oils start to set.

Scar Vanishing Cream

Ingredients:

    3 drops Melrose EO (for disinfecting scrapes, cuts or abrasions)

    3 drops Frankincense EO

    6 drops Lavender EO

    8 drops Lemongrass EO

    10 drops Geranium EO

    1 oz. Coconut Oil

Directions:

1. Heat Coconut oil in a glass bowl placed in a pot of simmering water or use a double broiler if you have one.

2. Remove the oil from heat once melted and transfer in a glass jar. Cool a bit. Once it's warm enough to touch, add all the essential oils. Stir thoroughly until all oils are incorporated.

3. This blend can be used in its liquid state or you can cool it in the refrigerator to set. Use it twice daily to reduce the appearance of your scar.

Honey Lemon Sugar Scrub

Ingredients:

¼ cup Olive Oil

1 cup Cane Sugar

2 tablespoons Honey

2 teaspoons dried Rosemary

15 drops Lavender EO

15 drops Lemon EO

Directions:

1. In a mixing bowl, combine sugar, honey, olive oil and dried rosemary.

2. Stir in the essential oils. Mix thoroughly until all ingredients are well combined.

3. Store in glass containers. This body scrub can last up to 3 months.

Cooling Peppermint Facial Toner

Ingredients:

¼ cup Apple Cider Vinegar

¾ cup Filtered Water

20 to 50 drops Peppermint Essential Oil

Directions:

1. Slowly mix apple cider vinegar and water. Pour into a glass spray bottle or any small glass bottle.

2. Add peppermint essential oil. Start by adding 20 drops. Test your toner before you add more peppermint EO. The more peppermint you add, the stronger is the cooling effect.

3. After cleansing your face in the morning and in the evening, lightly mist your face with this toner. You can also moisten a cotton ball with this toner and apply it on your face.

4. Store in the refrigerator when not in use.

Essential Oil Facial Serum

Ingredients:

　　1 oz Avocado Oil (or any carrier oil of your choice)

　　1 drop Rose EO

　　2 drops Frankincense EO

　　2 drops Sandalwood EO

Directions:

1. Place essential oils in a 1 ounce amber bottle with glass dropper.

2. Add avocado oil or any carrier oil of your choice.

3. Cover the bottle tightly and move it in an upward downward motion to mix all the oils.

4. Place 2 to 3 drops in a cotton ball and apply on face.

Chapter 3   Essential Oil Recipes For Home Use

Essential oils are also great for household use. Due to their great aroma, essential oils are often used to keep one's household smelling fresh and clean. Read on to find out more essential oil recipes for household use.

Air Freshener Blends

Ingredients:

2 drops Rose EO

4 drops Ylang Ylang EO

14 drops Bergamot EO

20 drops Lime EO

OR

6 drops Lavender EO

9 drops Lemon EO

15 drops Clary Sage EO

OR

2 drops Spearmint EO

4 drops Peppermint EO

8 drops Grapefruit EO

20 drops Rosemary EO

Directions:

1. Combine the essential oils in a (new, not used) spray bottle with 1.5 fl oz distilled water and 1.5 fl oz Vodka or Everclear.

2. Shake the bottle before each use to prevent oils from gathering on top of the mixture. You may add more essential oils if you think the scent is too weak or decrease the number of drops if you are sensitive to scents.

3. Be careful not to spray on beverages and furniture.

Carpet Deodorizer

Ingredients:

16 oz. Baking Soda

10 drops Lemon EO

20 drops Lavender EO

Directions:

1. Place baking soda in a mixing bowl.

2. Mix the essential oils until fully incorporated into the baking soda.

3. You may use your essential oil of choice for this recipe. Store in an airtight container.

4. Sprinkle deodorizer on your carpet and leave for 10 to 20 minutes. Vacuum your carpet normally.

Chapter 4   Aromatherapy Perfume Recipes

Since essential oils have natural scents, they are also great for perfumes. Furthermore, their therapeutic properties are also helpful for various situations. Check out the aromatherapy perfume recipes below and start blending your own perfumes.

Basic Perfume

Ingredients:

1 tablespoon Jojoba Oil

3 drops Jasmine Essential Oil (you may also use Rose or Neroli)

9 drops Sandalwood Essential Oil

Directions:

Blend them together in a dark, air-tight container. Dab a few drops on your pulse points as often as necessary.

Composure Perfume

Ingredients:

1 drop Coriander Essential Oil

2 drops Basil Essential Oil

3 drops Bergamot Essential Oil

4 drops Petitgrain Essential Oil

1 teaspoon Jojoba Oil

1 teaspoon Vodka

Directions:

1. Put 1 teaspoon Jojoba oil and 1 teaspoon Vodka in a dark glass container with an air-tight lid.

2. Add the essential oils, one drop at a time using a dropper.

3. Shake well after adding each essential oil.

4. Keep container tightly closed and store in a dark, cool area for 12 days. Shake mixture 3 times a day.

5. Do a skin patch test before using.

Essential Oil Cologne Blend For Men

Ingredients:

2 drops Neroli Essential Oils

3 drops Ginger Essential Oil

5 drops Oakmoss Absolute Essential Oil

5 drops Bay Laurel Essential Oil

15 drops Mandarin Essential Oil

15 drops Patchouli Essential Oil

1 fl oz Distilled Water

1.5 fl oz High Proof Vodka

Directions:

1. Put alcohol in a clean, glass container with a sprayer top. Add water and essential oils.

2. Shake vigorously until all oils are incorporated.

3. Let sit in a cool, dark area for 7 to 12 days. Shake the mixture 3 times a day for the oils to blend and mellow out.

4. Shake cologne before every use.

Confidence Blend

Ingredients:

2 drops Ginger Essential Oil

3 drops Verbena Essential Oil

3 drops Myrtle Essential Oil

4 drops Rosemary Essential Oil

Directions:

1. Combine 1 teaspoon Vodka and 1 teaspoon Jojoba Oil in a glass container with air-tight lid or cover.

2. Add essential oils, one drop at a time. Shake mixture after adding each drop of essential oil.

3. Cover and shake vigorously to incorporate all the ingredients.

4. Store in a dark, clean, cool area for 12 days while shaking 3 times each day.

5. Do not forget to do a patch test before using it regularly.

Aromatherapy Perfume For Moms

Ingredients:

4 drops Rose Essential Oil

3 drops Patchouli Essential Oil

3 drops Neroli Essential Oil

Directions:

1. Mix 1 teaspoon Jojoba Oil and 1 teaspoon Vodka in a glass container.

2. Add essential oils and shake vigorously.

3. Let the mixture stand for 12 days in a cool, dark area. Make sure to shake the bottle 3 times a day.

4. Essential oils may cause skin irritation so it is best to do a skin patch test first before using.

Chapter 5 Essential Oils For Emotions

Each essential oil has a unique scent and each also offers various benefits. Below is a guide to help you in choosing the right blend of essential oils for your needs.

Black Pepper Essential Oil – Stimulates and boosts energy.

Bergamot Essential Oil – Calms and uplifts the mind and body.

Cypress Essential Oil – Helps you feel secure, grounding.

Geranium Essential Oil – Uplifts the mind and body. Helps release nervous tension and get over negative memories.

Jasmine Essential Oil – Uplifts and relaxes the body.

Lavender Essential Oil – Relieves stress, promotes relaxation and helps reduce mental stress. Also promotes natural healing of cuts, scrapes and wounds.

Lemon Essential Oil – Boosts immunity and enhances focus.

Marjoram Essential Oil – Also known as the Herb of Happiness. Marjoram EO boosts the nervous system.

Melissa/Lemon Balm Essential Oil – Helps relieve stress and sleeplessness. It also helps release various emotions of the heart.

Neroli Absolute – Relaxes and uplifts the body and mind. For staying present.

Orange Essential Oil – Combats stress, boosts immunity, helps elevate the mind and body and brings peace and joy.

Patchouli Essential Oil- Relaxing and calming. Supports the nervous system and minimizes stress.

Roman Chamomile Essential Oil - Helps relieve sleeplessness and restlessness.

Rosemary Essential Oil – Helps reduce stress and enhances mental awareness.

Sandalwood Essential Oil – Boosts the nervous system.

Thyme Essential Oil – Helps release fear, balances emotions.

Valerian Essential Oil – Balances emotions, relaxing and grounding.

Vetiver Essential Oil – Grounding

Ylang-Ylang Essential Oil – Balances energies and restores confidence and peace.

Chapter 6 Essential Oils For Minor Aches/Pain

Balsam Fir Essential Oil – Helps ground the body and empower the mind. It also relaxes, soothes and warms the muscles.

Wintergreen Essential Oil – It contains Methyl Salicylate which soothes sore, tired muscles and head tension.

Birch Essential Oil – Also contains Methyl Salicylate. It warms and soothes the body emotionally, which helps greatly when going through any kind of discomfort.

Copaiba Essential Oil – Helps reduce irritation and discomfort due to muscle stiffness.

Roman Chamomile Essential Oil – Not only is this essential oil soothing to the skin, it is also great in relieving muscle discomfort especially after exercise.

Chapter 7 Essential Oils For Minor First Aid Needs

For disinfecting:

Hyssop Essential Oil

Melrose Essential Oil

Oregano Essential Oil

Tea Tree Essential Oil

Thieves Essential Oil

To help reduce bleeding:

Geranium Essential Oil

Helichrysum Essential Oil

Rose Otto Essential Oil

For infected wounds (antiseptic):

Clove Essential Oil

Elemi Essential Oil

Melrose Essential Oil

Myrrh Essential Oil

To promote natural healing:

Canadian Hemlock/Tsuga Essential Oil

Dorado Azul Essential Oil

Melrose Essential Oil

Purification Essential Oil

Tea Tree Essential Oil

To help reduce/vanish scarring:

Cistus Essential Oil

Geranium Essential Oil

Lavender Essential Oil

Chapter 8 Essential Oils For Insect Bites

The following oils have anti-bacterial, anti-infectious and anti-viral properties that are helpful in relieving tick bites:

Clove Essential Oil

Cypress Essential Oil

Exodus II Essential Oil

Melissa Essential Oil

Melrose Essential Oil

Oregano Essential Oil

Thieves Essential Oil

Thyme Essential Oil

If the tick is still attached, just put two drops directly on it and it will release its grip. To relieve itch, add 1 to 2 drops of these essential oils in the affected area.

The following essential oils are great for relieving Chigger bites.

Lavender Essential Oil

Tea Tree Essential Oil

Thieves Essential Oil

Thyme Essential Oil

Dilute essential oils in alcohol and apply directly on the affected area as needed or you may put 1 to 2 drops of essential oil on the insect bite. You may add 1 teaspoon of alcohol on ten drops of Thyme essential oil to relieve itchiness quickly. You may also place this mixture in a sprayer and use it as an insect repellant.

These essential oils quickly relieve itchiness and swelling due to gnat bites.

Lavender Essential Oil

Lemon Essential Oil

Purification Essential Oil

Thyme Essential Oil

You may apply 1 to 2 drops directly on the insect bite or you can mix 3 drops of Thyme essential oil in 1 tablespoon lemon juice or apple cider vinegar. Apply mixture on the affected area up to four times a day.

Spider bites can be dangerous but you can use essential oils to soothe the irritation. You can choose from the following or make your own blend:

1 drop Lavender Essential Oil

1 drop Melrose Essential Oil

1 drop Wintergreen Essential Oil

You need to consult a doctor afterwards. Apply essential oils on the insect bite every 10 minutes until you are treated by a physician.

Dilute essential oils in one tablespoon alcohol and apply on the affected area as required. You can choose from the following or make your own blend.

Fire ant bites hurt because they sting and inject venom directly into the skin. But, no worries, all you need is 1 to 2 drops of Purification essential oil applied on the bite and the swelling and itchiness will be relieved quickly. Apply as needed or up to 4 times a day. You can also use the following essential oils:

Basil Essential Oil

Lavender Essential Oil

Lemongrass Essential Oil

Thieves Essential Oil

Thyme Essential Oil

Mosquito bites can be very itchy and irritating. To soothe mosquito bites, you can use these essential oils:

Helichrysum Essential Oil

Lavender Essential Oil

Purification Essential Oil

You can either apply these oils directly on the bite or make your own blend.

Chapter 9 Essential Oils For Massage

Each essential oil has various properties. Blend these essential oils according to your needs. You can blend these essential oils to any carrier oil and use it for massage.

Ginger Essential Oil – Due to its warming effect, ginger essential oil is great for massage. It relaxes and soothes the muscles. It is also strengthening and anchoring.

Jasmine Absolute – Jasmine essential oil has a sweet, honey-like scent. It is very calm and relaxing, making it a great massage oil.

Lavender Essential Oil – Lavender essential oil has a sweet floral aroma that is very relaxing, calming and soothing. It also has healing properties making it a very good massage oil especially when blended with other essential oils.

Neroli Essential Oil – its strong, flowery, spicy aroma is very soothing and calming. It blends well with floral oils and citrus oils.

Oregano Essential Oil – This essential oil is very invigorating, uplifting and purifying. It is great for relieving stress and uplifting mood.

Peppermint Essential Oil – Its sweet, menthol aroma is refreshing, cooling and vitalizing.

Rosewood Essential Oil – It has a sweet, floral, woody aroma that gently strengthens and calms the body making it a great massage oil.

Sandalwood – Sandalwood essential oil is sensual, centering and relaxing. It blends well with most essential oils and is a common addition to massage oils.

Spearmint Essential Oil – This essential oil is often used to energize, refresh and vitalize the mind and body.

Vanilla Essential Oil – Its sweet balsamic aroma is comforting, balancing and calming.

Ylang-Ylang Essential Oil – It has a sweet, intense, floral aroma that makes it very sensual and euphoric. Best when blended with other floral-scented essential oils for massage.

Chapter 10 Essential Oils For Your Other Applications For Your Home

Lemon Essential Oil

Lemon is known for its antiseptic and anti-bacterial properties. It is also a great deodorizer and disinfectant. To remove gum, crayons, grease spots or oil, just place 1 to 2 drops directly to the area. To sterilize your countertops, add 2 to 3 drops of lemon essential oil to 1 liter of water and use it to spray the area. For fresh smelling utensils and plates, just add a drop or two on your dishwasher.

Eucalyptus Essential Oil

This essential oil is great for keeping your bathroom fresh and purified. Add 5 drops of Eucalyptus essential oil into the commode area for a fresh-smelling bathroom. To clean stainless steel items, add a few drops of eucalyptus essential oil on cloth and use it to rub on the item. To remove decals, stickers from glass, pour eucalyptus essential oil directly on them and leave for a few seconds and scrub off. To revive your old hanging car freshener, just add a few drops of eucalyptus essential oil.

Peppermint Essential Oil

This essential oil is great for putting the mice away. Put a few drops of Peppermint essential oil in water and place on a spray bottle. Use it to spray the areas where mice are staying. You can also put a few drops of peppermint essential oil in cotton balls and place them on your closet.

Conclusion

Our ancestors have traditionally used essential oils for many purposes. In today's modern time, living naturally is the best way to keep a healthy life and body.

Essential oils are readily available in the market. Using this book as a guide, you can make your own essential oil blends for many purposes. For many, essential oils are expensive. But, if you do the Math, you only use a few drops per blend and each blend lasts for months. Compare it to your commercially-made products and you will see the difference.

Furthermore, essential oils come from natural sources and are extracted using natural means such as by distillation. That is why essential oils are pure and very potent. Just a few drops go a long, long way. If you want to go green and stay away from chemically-laced products, using essential oils for your everyday needs is a must. Just be careful with people who are saying that essential oils can be taken internally.

This method is not yet proven and it can cause harm. Remember, essential oils are pure and concentrated. It is best to consult your physician before trying to take it internally.

This book provides essential oil recipes for various uses and a guide on the properties, aroma and benefits of each essential oil. You will now be able to concoct your own essential oil blend for your family and friends.

Enjoy this book?

Please leave a review below and let us know what you liked about this book.